Body Scrubs

The Complete Guide to Body Scrub Recipes and Uses

Robert S. Lee

Contents

Chapter 1. Body Scrubs & Using Them as Gifts

Body scrubs are meant to make a person feel wonderful, and if you do them right that's exactly what they can do. You can make someone feel wonderful through the flowers you use, scents, bases, and just the way it makes a person's skin feel soft, refreshed, and generally clean.

They remove a dead layer of cells on the surface of your skin, which helps people to look younger by revealing the younger cells beneath. Your skin, after a proper body scrub, will feel smooth and soft, and it has natural oils that will help to moisturize your skin to keep it from drying out. From essential oils and flowers with aromatherapy properties to bases, you can get people in a romantic mood, energize them, soothe them, or just relax them, depending on who you're giving your gift to and how you structure your body scrub.

Why Use It as a Gift?

Everyone wants to know what type of gift to give someone, and it can be so difficult to find something to give people that means anything. The countless gifts that are lining the shelves of various stores usually don't hold any meaning. When you make your own gift, then it has more meaning to you and the person you're giving it to, and body scrubs are easy to make. An easy, meaningful gift is always a good option.

Body scrubs are also extremely easy to make sure that they're specialized. You'll be able to make sure that you customize your gifts from the way you decorate them. You can choose a scent that means something to them, a scent that matches them, add a poem, or add their favorite color. Body scrubs are easy to make and personalize to fit your needs, and you're providing them with something that is both useful and luxurious.

Chapter 2. The Needed Supplies & Presentation Tips

You're going to have to prepare for making body scrubs, and the presentation really matters as well if you're giving them as a gift, so make sure that you have everything before you start. You're going to need these basic ingredients to get started.

Brown Sugar: Brown sugar is a great way to add a little more depth to your body scrub, and it's great if you're giving it to someone who likes something sweet. Of course, it's still coarse enough that you'll be able to exfoliate skin easily, and you don't need to add a lot of scents to it.

White Sugar: White sugar is used in a lot more body scrub recipes because it's a little more versatile.

Coarse Sea Salt: Sometimes, you don't want sugar, especially if you're trying to make something that smells a little manlier. To have a base that exfoliates skin, you're going to want salt. You can use table salt, but it's a lot finer, and doesn't work quite as well. Many people prefer coarse sea salt, but you can choose grain of your choice if you'd rather something a little smoother.

Olive Oil: Olive oil is an easy and cheap moisturizer to add to your body scrubs, and many different body scrub recipes will call for it. Of course, it's still good for your skin, and extremely healthy. It can make your skin look that much younger. Olive oil is even able to help with extremely dry skin.

Sweet Almond Oil: Sweet almond oil can help you to treat different rashes, skin irritations, and even acne. It's great for your skin, and goes well into a body scrub. You'll find that it helps to make sure that you have everything you need to moisturize skin as well. It can even remove dark spots, and is great for anti-aging.

Essential Oils: Make sure you have therapeutic grade essential oils if you want to use them in a body scrub for their abilities more than just their scents. However, if you're just looking for a scent, a cheaper grade could work. Some of the best essential oils to keep on hand is cedarwood, sandalwood, orange blossom, rose, and lavender. This gives you a balance, and essential oils can always be substituted to create a slightly different body scrub.

A Glass Jar: You're going to need an airtight glass jar. The colorful look of your body scrub is part of the appeal, so glass jars are a must. Make sure it's airtight, and many people will use mason jars. You can even decorate the top rather easily.

Presentation Tips:

If you're giving something as a gift, presentation always matter. This doesn't change with body scrubs. The body scrub you choose will also depend on how you decorate it, but there are many tips for creating an easy and beautiful body scrub that you're still able to personalize.

Cardstock for Tags is a Must: A heavy duty paper like cardstock is always important to have so you can print or write tags. It can tell them the name of the scrub, a description, or just the ingredients and directions. Most people don't need direction with a body scrub, so put something a little more personal on it, and you can get different colors and designs of this heavy duty paper to make a tag that makes it great for a gift.

Lace or Ribbon Sets it Off: Lace or ribbon is important because it will allow you to tie the tag around the jar, and it'll help to make sure that your tag stays on and add a little more presentation to it. Make sure to have a large variety, but it doesn't have to necessarily be expensive.

Cloth Squares Help to Personalize: You're always going to want a homemade touch to what you're making, and a tag is a great place to start, but having cloth squares helps as well. You can get these at any fabric store, and they're not that hard. Or, if you're making a lot of them you can always get a large amount of cloth and trim it down to the size you need. Just hot glue it to the top of the jar, and sometimes put some cotton balls underneath to give it a plush look that gives it a rounded top. It's completely up to you. Using hot glue will keep it on, and make it a little prettier. You can even use a specialized pair of scissors to cut a pattern at the bottom.

Chapter 3. Body Scrubs for Anti-Aging & Wrinkles

Sometimes you know older people who are a little worried about wrinkles, dark spots, and the general effects of aging. Everybody scrub helps to make your skin look a little better, healthier, and even younger, but some are specialized to help make sure that you're dealing with wrinkles and the process of aging. These make great gifts to an aging friend who's worried about it, but never give it to someone who might get insulted by it. You can eve use it to help with the effects of aging yourself. These body scrubs can double as a facemask.

Body Scrub #1 Pumpkin & Sugar Scrub

This pumpkin scrub is great for anyone who loves a natural touch, and it's great for anti-aging. Pumpkin puree is known to be anti-aging because of the antioxidant levels, and the exfoliation provided by a sugar scrub helps with aging in the first place. The honey also provides your face a bit of an uplift, helps with acne, and is even known to help with wrinkles.

Ingredients:

1. 1 Tablespoon Honey, Raw
2. 1 Tablespoon Olive Oil
3. ½ Cup Brown Sugar, Light & Packed
4. ½ Cup Pumpkin Puree, No Added Sugar

Directions:

1. Mix all ingredients together. Make sure they're thoroughly mixed, but do not overly mix if you do not want it to

become too fine. If you want it to be thicker, add a little more brown sugar.

Body Scrub #2 Oatmeal & Honey Scrub

Honey, as stated before, is really great for your skin, and you'll find due to the antioxidant amounts it's great for anti-aging. Oatmeal is also an anti-inflammatory and full of antioxidants, which are two things that are helpful when dealing with the effects of aging. It can even relieve skin irritations. Almond oil is a light oil that isn't greasy, so it's less likely to cause any acne, and it's great at moisturizing your skin.

Ingredients:

1. ¼ Cup Honey, Raw
2. ½ Cup Oats, Raw
3. ¼ Cup Sweet Almond Oil

Directions:

1. Mix everything together, and do not blend unless desired for a thinner consistency. Of course, add more oats if you want the mixture to be thicker.

Body Scrub #3 Sweet Lemon Body Scrub

Lemon essential oil is great for making sure that dark spots start to disappear, and it can even help with wrinkles. The almond oil is meant to nourish your skin, making it look smoother and younger. The honey is full of antioxidants that will help with aging, and white sugar will help to make it sweet and exfoliate.

Ingredients:

1. 1 Cup White Sugar
2. ¼ Cup Honey, Raw
3. 2 Tablespoons Sweet Almond Oil
4. 10-15 Drops Lemon Essential Oil

Directions:

1. Mix everything together, and if it is too thick, add more almond oil. If too thin, add more sugar.

Body Scrub #4 Nutmeg & Ginger Sugar Scrub

Nutmeg essential oil helps with premature aging, and ginger is a great anti-inflammatory which will help with the effects of aging as well.

It's an easy and simple sugar scrub recipe that's quite fragrant.

Ingredients:

1. 1 Cup White Sugar
2. ½ Cup Coconut Oil, Melted
3. 10-12 Drops Nutmeg Essential Oil
4. 4-6 Drops Ginger Essential Oil

Directions:

1. Mix all ingredients together before placing into a jar to decorate later.

Chapter 4. Flower Body Scrub Recipes

This is a much wider category of body scrubs, and it works better for gifts because it applies to more people. There are many different flowers that can be added, and they have different effects as well. They're great for women, and they're very fragrant.

Body Scrub #5 Rose Sugar Scrub

Roses are a common flower to use, and you can get rose petals from a store or use one that you grow yourself. Of course, make sure your petals are fragrant, as sometimes when you buy them they may not be. Bruised petals always provide more scent, and you can lightly bruise them with your fingers before adding them in. Of course, this is a recipe that calls for dried rose petals. You can substitute for fresh if desired.

Ingredients:

1. 6-9 Drops Vanilla Essential Oil
2. 2/3 Cup Sweet Almond Oil
3. 2 Cups White Sugar
4. 1 Cup Rose Petals, Dried

Directions:

1. Take your rose petals, and blend them lightly in a food processor until they become beautiful but small flakes. The size is up to you.
2. Add all another ingredients together, and then lightly mix the rose petals in. for presentation, you can add a small layer of petals on top and bottom as well.

Body Scrub #6 Lavender Salt Scrub

Lavender is yet another floral scent that is wonderful and beautiful. You get a light lilac color, but it's mostly white. Many people prefer to add the fresh petals on top and bottom for presentation, and it's a relaxing salt scrub. Germanium essential oil is meant to help with uplifting your mood, and it helps to calm the spirit and mind.

Ingredients:

1. 1 Cup Sea Salt, Coarse
2. ½ Cup Sweet Almond Oil
3. ¼ Cup Lavender Buds, Dried
4. ¼ Teaspoon (6-8 Drops) Geranium Essential Oil
5. ¼ Cup Fresh Lavender Petals

Directions:

1. Mix all ingredients expect the fresh petals together, and make sure it's mixed completely.
2. Place half the fresh flowers on the bottom of the jar, spooning in the rest of the mixture, and topping it with the last half of the fresh flowers

Body Scrub #7 Rose & Chamomile Body Scrub

This doubles as a face scrub, like most sugar scrubs, and the chamomile is meant to be relaxing. Chamomile is also meant to sooth dry and irritated skin, which is a great addition to any body scrub.

Ingredients:

1. 2 Tablespoons Honey, Raw
2. ½ Sweet Almond Oil
3. 1 Cup Sea Salt, Coarse

4. 2 Tablespoons Oats, Raw
5. 2 Tablespoons Rose Petals, Dried
6. 2 Tablespoons Chamomile Flowers, Dried

Directions:

1. Just mix everything together, not blending anything. Break apart the rose petals first if you want them to be smaller. Place into jars, and decorate as you please.

Body Scrub #8 Chamomile Body Scrub

This is a wonderful rosemary and chamomile sugar scrub that is sure to calm your mind and body. It helps your skin to look younger, and it's easy to make. Rosemary gives it a more earthy scent to it, and you can even add a little rosemary essential oil to stabilize your mood.

Ingredients:

1. 10-15 Drops Rosemary Essential Oil
2. 2 Cups White Sugar
3. ¼ Cup Chamomile Flowers, Dried
4. 1 Cup Sweet Almond Oil
5. 1 Teaspoon Rosemary, Dried

Directions:

1. Mix all ingredients together, and it should give your body scrub a flowery and very distinct smell.

Body Scrub #9 Orange & Rose Scrub

Oranges are a light and fruity scent that pairs well with roses, and this one has a bit of color added into it because of the ground rose petals and the ground orange zest. You can even dry your own orange peel and grind it in a food processor or by hand.

Ingredients:

1. 2 Tablespoons Honey, Raw
2. ½ Cup Sweet Almond Oil
3. ½ Cup Coconut Oil
4. 1 Cup Rose Petals, Dried
5. 2 Tablespoons Rose Petals, Dried
6. 1 Tablespoon Orange Zest, Dried
7. 1 Cup White Sugar

Directions:

1. Blend the two tablespoons of rose petals and orange zest together, and mix it with the coconut oil, sweet almond oil, and rose petals. It should give it a light pink color. Add in the honey, and continue to mix.

2. Divide your cup of dried rose petals into three. Put one layer on the bottom, spoon in the mixture, add another layer,

spoon in the mixture, and then add more rose petals to top.

Body Scrub #10 Lavender & Lemon Scrub

The vanilla essential oil gives it a more even tone to it, and you'll find that the lavender flowers give it a beautiful look when you're packaging it for a gift. Of course, the lemon zest and lavender blending together and being added to the salt helps to make sure that you have a beautiful and colorful salt scrub.

Ingredients:

1. 1 Cup Sea Salt, Coarse
2. 1 Cup Lavender Flowers, Dried& Divided
3. 4-5 Drops Vanilla Essential Oil
4. ½ Cup Sweet Almond Oil
5. 3 Tablespoons Lemon Zest

Directions:

1. Take a food processor, blending a half a cup of the lavender flowers and lemon zest, mixing it together.
2. Mix it into sea salt, sweet almond oil, and vanilla essential oil. Mix by hand.
3. Layer the bottom, top and middle with the remaining lavender flowers. Put the sugar scrub in between. You can sprinkle on more lemon zest if desired.

Chapter 5. More Manly Recipes as Gifts

Sometimes you don't want something that has too much fruity or flowering scents when you're trying to use a body scrub as a gift for a man. So you'll find that it'll help to have some more manly scented recipes that don't involve flowers as heavily.

Recipe #11 Green Tea & Eucalyptus Scrub

Eucalyptus is a relaxing scent without it being too feminine. The green tea is also great for your skin, and it's a mild stimulant. This isn't an overpowering smell, but you can add more eucalyptus oil if desired. The sugar and salt act as excellent exfoliates together.

25

Ingredients:

1. ½ Cup Olive Oil
2. ¼ Cup Sea Salt, Coarse
3. ¾ Cup White Sugar
4. ½ Tablespoon Matcha Green Tea Powder
5. ½ Teaspoon Eucalyptus Essential Oil

Directions:

1. Just mix all of your ingredients together before storing in a jar. Decorate as desired.

Recipe #12 Perky Sugar & Salt Scrub

The coffee grounds help to give this a wonderful and unique body scrub that has a unique scent to it. You'll be able to give your man a wonderful body scrub that doesn't seem girly. It isn't even girly in color.

Ingredients:

1. 1 Cup White Sugar
2. ½ Cup Coarse Sea Salt
3. ¼ Cup Coffee Grounds
4. 8-12 Drops Vanilla Essential Oil
5. 5-7 Drops Peppermint Essential Oil
6. 1/3 Cup Olive Oil

Directions:

1. Mix all ingredients together, and then place into a jar with an airtight container.

Recipe #13 Rugged Lemon Body Scrub

Lemon is a rather universal scent, and it isn't too girly, making it perfect for a scrub that you're giving a man. You can use a full cup of sea salt if preferred, and it's great for tough hands. If you want it to be thicker, just add more salt. The essential oil helps to make sure the lemon scent is prominent, but the lemon zest gives it a beautiful yellow color that isn't too bright.

Ingredients:

1. ½ Cups White Sugar
2. ½ Cup Sea Salt, Coarse

3. ½ Cup Olive Oil
4. 2 Tablespoons Lemon Zest
5. 3-5 Drops Lemon Essential Oil

Directions:

1. Blend everything together and put into a jar. It should have a prominent lemon scent.

Recipe #14 Sage & Sandalwood Scrub

Sage and sandalwood are both manly scents that work extremely well together, and the sage gives a bit of a wonderful texture to it. You can get it right from your kitchen cabinet, and sandalwood essential oil is an anti-inflammatory and astringent. It's even slightly calming.

Ingredients:

1. 10-12 Drops Sandalwood Essential Oil
2. ½ Cup Sea Salt, Coarse
3. ½ Cup White Sugar
4. 2 Tablespoons Sage, Ground
5. ½ Cup Olive Oil

Directions:

1. Blend everything together, and then place it in an airtight glass jar. Decorate as desired.

Recipe #15 Pine Body Scrub

Pine is known to be a manly scent, and with olive oil, you get the right green tinge to your body scrub that you need. Of course, make sure not to go overboard on the decorating if you want it to stay looking manly. It's very aromatic, and it's a great stimulating scent that will give anyone a pick me up.

Ingredients:

1. 1 Cup Sea Salt, Medium to Coarse
2. 15-20 Drops Essential Oil
3. ½ Cup Olive Oil

Directions:

1. Just mix everything together, and then put it into a jar before decorating it.

Recipe #16 Sage & Clove Scrub

Sage is a great scent, and it's easy to give a texture to your salt and sugar scrub. The cloves and sage together make a wonderful scent, and clove oil is meant to relax you and relieve stress. Men deal with built up stress like everyone else, even if they don't always want to admit it.

Ingredients:

1. ½ Cup Sea Salt, Coarse
2. ½ Cup White Sugar
3. 10-15 Drops Clove Essential Oil
4. 3 Tablespoons Sage, Dried
5. ½ Cup Olive Oil

Directions:

1. Just mix everything together. Blend the sage smaller if you need it to be, and place in an airtight glass container for storage.

Recipe #17 Cedar Wood Scrub

The cedarwood is a great essential oil, and it has a manly scent. It is meant to calm you down, give you peace of mind, and it even helps to make sure that you're relaxed and it is a great astringent. The sweet almond oil provides moisturizing effects that soothes skin, and it gives another layer of depth to the scent and the scrub.

Ingredients:

1. ½ Cup Sea Salt, Coarse
2. ½ Cup White Sugar
3. 15-20 Drops Cedarwood Essential Oil
4. ½ Sweet Almond Oil

Directions:

1. Mix all ingredients together, and then place it in a jar and decorate as desired. It will not have a dark look without the olive oil, but sweet almond oil works best for the scent.

Recipe #18 Cypress & Sandal Wood Scrub

Cypress essential oil is an astringent, and it's able to sooth inflammation as well as remove body odor. It's great at soothing inflammation as well. Sandalwood is also an anti-inflammatory, an astringent, and it is great for increasing your memory and helping with anxiety and stress.

Ingredients:

1. 1 Cup Sea Salt, Medium to Coarse
2. ½ Cup Olive Oil
3. 10-12 Drops Cypress Essential Oil
4. 15-20 Drops Sandalwood Essential Oil

Directions:

1. Mix everything together, and then put it in a glass jar and seal tight for storage.

Chapter 6. Holiday Themed Body Scrubs to Try

There are many holidays that you'll end up needing a gift for, and body scrubs can still be that gift. If you don't know how to personalize them to the person, you can always personalize them to the holiday. There are many colors and scents related to different holidays, and it's a great theme to stick with.

Recipe #19 A Peppermint Christmas Scrub

Peppermint is known to be a very Christmas like scent, and it's easy to get into a body scrub. You can keep it white if you want, but there are ways to decorate it up with reds. This sugar scrub is green, as it's a lighter food coloring and much less likely to stain. Peppermint is also a soothing and rejuvenating scent. You can use a half a teaspoon of peppermint extract in a pinch if you don't have peppermint essential oil on hand.

Ingredients:

1. 1 Cup White Sugar
2. 1/3 Cup Sweet Almond Oil
3. 10-15 Drops Peppermint Essential Oil
4. 2 Tablespoons Honey, Raw
5. 1 Drop Green Food Coloring

Directions:

1. Mix everything together, and add more sugar if you need it to be thicker. Decorate as desired. If you have a food coloring you know will not dye, you can

make two batches or cut this one in half, mixing one half with red and one half with green. You can then layer it for an added effect.

Recipe #20 Gingerbread Sugar Scrub

Gingerbread is also a well-known scent around Christmas, and you can even make a gingerbread man tag if you want to make sure that it's really Christmas like. This makes one and a quarter cups. Vanilla essential oil is full of antioxidants that allows your skin to get a healthy glow, and nutmeg essential oil is added because it is known to counter aging.

Ingredients:

1. ¼ Teaspoon Cinnamon, Ground
2. 2-4 Drops Nutmeg Essential Oil
3. ¼ Teaspoon Ginger, Ground
4. ¼ Teaspoon Allspice, Ground

5. 4-6 Drops Vanilla Essential Oil
6. ½ Cup White Sugar
7. ½ Cup Brown Sugar, Light
8. ¾ Cup Sweet Almond Oil

Directions:

1. Blend everything together before putting it into the jar. If too thin, then add a little more brown sugar until the right consistency is reached.

Recipe #21 Vanilla & Rose Scrub

Vanilla and roses are great scents for Valentine's Day, and it has just a light pink color if you're mixing in powdered rose petals as well. It's easy to make, and vanilla essential oil gives it a powerful and relaxing scent. Adding some salt will make it a little coarser, which boosts its exfoliating properties, helping your skin to be even smoother.

Ingredients:

1. 1 Cup Rose Petals, Dried
2. 2 Tablespoons Rose Petals, Dried
3. 2 Teaspoons Sea Salt, Coarse
4. 5-8 Drops Vanilla Essential Oil
5. 1 Cup White Sugar

Direction:

1. Start by blending your two tablespoons rose petals and sea salt together.
2. Add the vanilla essential oils and sugar to the blended salt mixture, giving your mix a little more color.
3. Layer the mixture in a glass jar between layers of rose petals for a sweet and romantic look.

Recipe #22 Pink Lemonade Scrub

This isn't as romantic as a rose scrub, but for Valentine's Day pink is the thing, and not every girl wants rose scented gifts. Of course, you'll find that it's an excellent pink color when you're finished, and it gives you a lot to decorate.

Ingredients:

1. 1 Drop Red Food Coloring
2. 1 Cup White Sugar
3. 5-8 Drops Lemon Essential Oil
4. ¼ Cup Sweet Almond Oil

Directions:

1. Mix everything together, and then add in the food coloring last. If you need it to be thicker, add more white sugar.

Recipe #23 Pumpkin Spice & Vanilla Scrub

Vanilla essential oil is both relaxing and calming. It's also a great mood stabilizer, and you'll find that the pumpkin pie spice gives you the smell of Halloween, making it a great gift. Of course, with cinnamon essential oil you have an added astringent.

Ingredients:

1. ½ Cup Sweet Almond Oil
2. 1 Cup White Sugar
3. ½ Teaspoon Pumpkin Pie Spice
4. 6-8 Drops Vanilla Essential Oil
5. 2-4 Drops Cinnamon Essential Oil

Directions:

1. Just mix everything together until it's mixed thoroughly, and then place it in an airtight container, decorating as desired.

Recipe #24 Chocolate & Coconut Sugar Scrub

If you like Easter, you know that there is usually chocolate involved. Coconut cake is also an Easter favorite, so you can mix the two in this wonderful Easter sugar scrub. It's easy to make, and fun to decorate. The coconut oil is just as moisturizing as sweet almond oil.

Ingredients:

1. 1 Cup Brown Sugar, Light
2. ½ Cup Coconut Oil
3. 2 Tablespoons Cocoa Powdered, Unsweetened

Directions:

1. Just mix everything together, and then put it into a glass jar and seal. Decorate in Easter colors.

Recipe #25 Cherry Blossoms Mother's Day Scrub

Cherry blossoms are a wonderful scent, and you can buy them dried. Of course, fresh cherry blossoms work as well. You'll find that the almond oil doesn't contribute to the scent too much, so cherry is still the main scent. It's a light color, and when you grind the cherry blossoms, then it'll give it a little extra color.

Ingredients:

1. 1 Cup White Sugar
2. ½ Cup Sweet Almond Oil
3. 1 Cup Cherry Blossom Petals, Dried
4. 2 Tablespoons Cherry Blossoms, Dried

Directions:

1. Start by grinding your two tablespoons cherry blossoms, and then mix it with sweet almond oil and white sugar.
2. Layer it in between dried cherry blossoms for the best presentation.

Chapter 7. Colored Ones to Dazzle Your Friends

If you are unsure of how to personalize your body scrubs, you can always go with various colors. It's easy to make sure that you get any color you want, so your body scrubs don't have to be plain. Instead, you can brighten the day with any color you like.

Recipe #26 Candy Blue Sugar Scrub

Make sure to get a light colored blue so it doesn't stain anything, but you'll have a candy like scent coming from this sugar scrub. It's great for anyone's inner child, and blue sugar scrubs are hard to get, so it'll be a unique gift that's still calming and great for your skin due to the vanilla essential oil and sweet almond oil.

Ingredients:

1. 1 Cup White Sugar
2. 4-6 Drops Vanilla Essential Oil
3. ½ Cup Sweet Almond Oil
4. 1 Package Blue Raspberry Drink Mix

Directions:

1. Mix everything together, and then place it in an airtight container before decorating.

Recipe #27 Mango Orange Body Scrub

Remember that this body scrub has to be kept refrigerated, but it's a nice orange color, even if you get a yellow mango which is a little less stringy, so it's recommended. Orange essential oil is known to help uplift your mood, fighting stress and depression, and it's even known as an anti-inflammatory, so it helps to soothe skin.

Ingredients:

1. ¼ Cup Yellow Mango, Cubed
2. 4-6 Drops Orange Essential Oil
3. 2 Tablespoons Sweet Almond Oil
4. ½ Cup White Sugar

Directions:

1. Blend the sweet almond oil and the yellow mango together.
2. Add everything else, and mix together, spooning into glass jars before sealing.

Recipe #28 Green Tea Sugar Scrub

Green tea is a great green color when you do it up right, and it has a refreshing smell that almost everyone loves. You won't need an essential oil for this one, and if you're looking for green tea leaves, you can always open up a green tea bag for a cheaper option. Green tea is also known to be great for your skin, and it has many antioxidants and anti-aging effects. It can also uplift your mood and energy levels.

Ingredients:

1. 2 Tablespoons Green Tea Leaves
2. 1 Cup White Sugar
3. ½ Cup Sweet Almond Oil
4. 2 Teaspoons Green Tea Powder

Directions:

1. Mix all ingredients together, and then place it in an airtight container. Glass is usually best, and it'll help to show off the color.

Recipe #29 Lemon & Thyme Yellow Scrub

When you think yellow, you usually think lemon, but lemon on its own isn't that original. Try lemon and thyme for an earthy and great scent that is neither manly nor girly. It's easy to make, and thyme is something that you can usually find in your kitchen cabinet.

Ingredients:

1. 2 Lemons, Fresh & Squeezed
2. ½ Tablespoon Olive Oil
3. 3 Tablespoons Thyme, Dried
4. 1 Cup White Sugar

Directions:

1. Mix the juice from your squeezed lemons in with all other ingredients. Make sure

that it's completely mixed, and then put it in an airtight glass container.
2. If you need to have it thicker, just add more sugar.

Recipe #30 Red Cherry Sugar Scrub

If you like cherries, then you'll love this sweet sugar scrub. It's great for almost anyone on your list. Of course, you can always use salt if you want it to be a little less sweet, but white sugar is known to work best. The sweet almond oil makes sure that your skin looks glowing and new in just a few uses. You can say goodbye to dead skin and hello to smooth, beautiful skin with a great smell. Cherry essential oil is known to help you feel calmer and in a better place mentally.

Ingredients:

1. ½ Cup Sweet Almond Oil

2. 4-5 Drops Cherry Essential Oil
3. 10 Drops Red Soap Colorant
4. 1 Cup White Sugar

Directions:

1. Mix everything together before placing in an airtight glass jar.

Recipe #31 Sleepy Time Blend

This purple body scrub is great for anyone on your list that needs a little more incentive to relax and loves the color purple. Roman chamomile essential oil is anti-inflammatory which helps with the aging process, it provides stress relief, helps to promote sleep, and has a calming effect on the mind. Vanilla essential oil is great at making sure that you have a sweet undertone that removes stress as well, along with the lavender essential oil that is added to go with the lavender buds.

Ingredients:

1. ½ Cup Lavender Buds, Dried
2. 2-4 Drops Lavender Essential Oil
3. 7-10 Drops Roman Chamomile Essential Oil
4. 4-5 Drops Vanilla Essential Oil
5. 4-5 Drops Purple Soap Colorant
6. 1 Cup White Sugar
7. ½ Cup Sweet Almond Oil

Directions:

1. Mix all your ingredients together except your lavender buds. Layer them in the jar between layers of the sugar scrub mixture.

Recipe #32 Rose & Rosemary Sugar Scrub

Pink is a lot lighter than red, and it's a beautiful color for a girly sugar scrub that is sure to leave your skin baby soft. Rose essential oil is known to fight depression and uplift your mood, and rosemary essential oil will help to fight inflammation, helping to make sure that you have everything you need to fight aging.

Ingredients:

1. 8-10 Drops Rose Essential Oil
2. ½ Cup Rose Petals, Dried
3. 5-6 Drops Rosemary Essential Oil
4. ½ Cup Sweet Almond Oil
5. 1 Cup White Sugar
6. 1-2 Drops Red Food Coloring

Directions:

1. Mix all ingredients together except the rose petals. Layer the scrub between layers of rose petals for decoration.

Chapter 8. Body Scrubs for Extra Uses

There are many ways to get softer skin and even have other benefits for your skin, like fighting of cellulite, from different body scrub recipes. They're fun and easy to make just like the others, and they are a great, useful and fragrant gift to give anyone on your list. There are many different essential oils used, and sweet almond oil already gives you a boost to your skin to make it glow as well as being a little healthier.

Body Scrub #33 Cellulite Fighter

Coconut oil, coffee grounds, and cinnamon essential oil is known to help tighten the skin and make it a little healthier, helping to fight cellulite. You'll find that with white sugar, it's a sweet sugar scrub that is great for everyone. Cinnamon wakes up the mind and centers you.

Ingredients:

1. ½ Cup Coconut Oil, Extra Virgin
2. 1 Cup Coffee Grounds
3. 1 Cup White Sugar
4. 6-8 Drops Cinnamon Essential Oil

Directions:

1. The coconut oil will give you bright and glowing skin, but make sure that it's melted. Add it with all other ingredients, making sure it's well mixed.

Body Scrub #34 Eczema Body Scrub

Lavender essential oil is antifungal, antibacterial and anti-inflammatory. The thyme is also known to help with eczema, and geranium. It's known to help with inflammation and kill any bacteria that can be harming your skin. Sweet almond oil is also good for dry skin, which helps with eczema.

Ingredients:

1. 1 Cup White Sugar
2. ½ Cup Sweet Almond Oil
3. 2 Tablespoons Thyme, Dried
4. 5-8 Drops Lavender Essential Oil
5. 10-12 Drops Geranium Essential Oil

Directions:

1. Mix everything together and then put it in an airtight glass container. Remember to decorate as desired before giving it as a gift.

Body Scrub #35 Psoriasis Body Scrub Help

Sandalwood essential oil is meant to make sure that your immune system is brought back into balance, which is known to help with psoriasis. Sweet almond oil helps to soothe the skin, and thyme essential oil is helpful to providing immediate relief. Remember that thyme essential oil must never be used on its own, as it is a skin irritant, and you need to make sure that it is not ingested as it is toxic. You should not use thyme essential oil if you are pregnant, breastfeeding, or if you have high blood pressure. Tea tree essential oil is great for a variety of skin problems, including psoriasis.

Ingredients:

1. ¾ Cup White Sugar
2. ¼ Cup Sea Salt, Fine
3. 1 Teaspoon Thyme, Dried
4. 4-6 Drops Thyme Essential Oil
5. 2-4 Drops Tea Tree Essential Oil
6. ¼ Cup Sweet Almond Oil
7. 8-10 Drops Sandalwood Essential Oil

Directions:

1. Just mix everything together and then put it in a glass jar so it's ready for decorating.

Body Scrub #36 Itchy Skin Relief Scrub

Coconut oil is already going to soothe your already itchy. Carrot seed oil has many skin healing abilities, as well as the ability to make your skin glow. It'll easily soothe irritated skin, as well as Roman chamomile. It's even a great relaxant, helping you to relax while your itchy skin becomes a thing of the past.

Ingredients:

1. 1 Cup White Sugar
2. ½ Cup Coconut Oil, Melted
3. 5-8 Drops Roman Chamomile Essential Oil
4. 4-6 Drops Carrot Seed Essential Oil

Directions:

1. Mix everything together, and add more coconut oil if needed.

Body Scrub #37 A Sunburn Body Scrub

If you're looking for a body scrub for sunburn, you're going to want to have it a little more liquid, as you don't want it to be quite as abrasive. That's one reason you'll want to use sugar as well. Aloe vera gel is great at making sure that you have everything you need to have your skin healed, rose petals are also known to soothe the burn, much like peppermint essential oil. The coconut oil is smooth and will provide the proper texture while giving you the vitamin E you need for your skin to heal up in a healthy manner.

Ingredients:

1. ½ Cup White Sugar
2. ½ Cup Aloe Vera Gel
3. ½ Cup Rose Petals, Fresh
4. ¼ Cup Coconut Oil, Extra Virgin
5. 5-6 Drops Peppermint Essential Oil

Directions:

1. Mix everything together after heating the aloe vera gel and coconut oil lightly in a double boiler together, making sure your rose petals are bruised. Let it sit for at least two days before using, and place in an airtight glass container. Decorate as desired.

Body Scrub #38 Another Eczema Relief Scrub

Helichrysum essential oil is great at soothing your skin and your mind, and it's an anti-allergenic, which helps with eczema as well as psoriasis. It even has pain reducing properties which will help immediately. Peppermint essential oil also provides some relief, especially paired with carrot seed essential oil which has skin healing abilities. With sweet almond oil to provide a soothing base, you'll find that this is a great eczema relief body scrub.

Ingredients:

1. ½ Cup Sweet Almond Oil
2. ¼ Cup Sea Salt, Fine
3. ¾ Cup White Sugar
4. 5-8 Drops Helichrysum Essential Oil
5. 4-5 Drops Peppermint Essential Oil
6. 8-10 Drops Carrot Seed Essential Oil

Directions:

1. Mix all ingredients together, and then place in an airtight glass container and save for decorating later.

Chapter 9. Body Scrub Recipes for Your Mood

There are many times in your life that you may suffer from stress, anxiety or depression which will dampen your mood. Of course, there are many different essential oils that will help to brighten your mood and fight your stress. When added into a body scrub you can have better skin and a better mood in no time, and it still can make the perfect gift.

Body Scrub #39 Jasmine & Bergamot

Jasmine is a flowery scent that is very uplifting, and it's great for relaxation. When paired with bergamot essential oil, you'll be able to relief anxiety, sadness and depression. It's also an uplifting scent, and it's a powerful duo when paired together in this wonderful, skin softening body scrub.

Ingredients:

1. ½ Cup Jasmine Flowers, Fresh
2. 10-15 Drops Jasmine Essential Oil
3. 8-10 Drops Bergamot Essential Oil
4. 1 Cup Sea Salt, Fine
5. ½ Cup Sweet Almond Oil

Directions:

1. Do not add the jasmine flowers in. Mix all other ingredients together, and then layer between jasmine flower layers.

Body Scrub #40 Chamomile & Sandalwood Scrub

This is an earthy and slightly flowery smelling body scrub that is sure to improve your mood and promote relaxation, including helping you with establishing a sleep cycle if you use it at night. It should be Roman chamomile, and you'll find that it is meant to relax both the mind and body. It's often been used to treat stress and depression, and when paired with Sandalwood's sedative properties, all your tension and stress should be relieved in this natural sugar body scrub.

Ingredients:

1. ¼ Cup Coconut Oil, Melted
2. ¼ Cup Sweet Almond Oil
3. ¼ Cup Sea Salt, Fine
4. ¾ Cup White Sugar
5. 10-15 Drops Roman Chamomile Essential Oil
6. 8-10 Drops Sandalwood Essential Oil

Directions:

1. Mix everything together, making sure that the essential oils are mixed evenly.

Body Scrub #41 Bergamot & Rose Sugar Scrub

Bergamot as said before is a great way relax, and it pairs so well with flowery scents. You'll find that rose is relaxing as well, but make sure you're getting a therapeutic grade of rose essential oil, and make sure you use it sparingly, as often they are little more expensive than other essential oils. Rose essential oil gives you a sense of well-being because it stimulates your entire nervous system.

Ingredients:

1. 8-10 Drops Bergamot Essential Oil
2. 10-15 Drops Rose Essential Oil
3. 1 Cup White Sugar

4. ½ Cup Sweet Almond Oil
5. ½ Cup Rose Petals, Dried

Directions:

1. Mix everything together except the rose petals. Layer the rose petals in between the layer of scrub for a better presentation.

Body Scrub #42 Sweet Wild Orange & Jasmine

Wild orange always pairs well with a flowery scent like jasmine, and it's sure to be relaxing with jasmine's relaxing and calming scent. When you add wild orange essential on top of it your stress and depression should start to melt away. Wild orange is known to energize you, lift your mood, and relieve nervousness. With sweet almond oil to make your skin glow and smooth, you have a body scrub that will be sure to please anyone you gift it to.

Ingredients:

1. 15-20 Drops Wild Orange Essential Oil
2. 8-10 Drops Jasmine Essential Oil
3. ½ Cup Sweet Almond Oil
4. 1 Cup White Sugar
5. ½ Cup Jasmine Flowers, Fresh

Directions:

1. Just mix all ingredients together, place it in a glass container and get ready to decorate.

Body Scrub #43 Marjoram & Clary Sage

Marjoram is great with clary sage, and if you want to add in a little more scent, add in dried jasmine or rose petals. Of course, clary sage essential oil is great for anxiety as well as depression. Of course, marjoram is great for anxiety, so you don't have to worry about anxiety and stress anymore.

Ingredients:

1. ½ Cup Sweet Almond Oil
2. 1 Cup White Sugar
3. 10-12 Drops Marjoram Essential Oil
4. 6-8 Drops Clary Sage Essential Oil

Directions:

1. Mix all of the ingredients together making sure the essential oil is completely mixed all the way through, and then put in an airtight glass container for storage. Remember to decorate as desired.

Chapter 10. Final Recipes & Tips for Body Scrub Gifts

Here are a few more recipes that you can use for the best body scrub gifts for anyone in the family. It'll work any friend, just know how to decorate and you'll be on your way to making the perfect homemade gift in no time.

Body Scrub #44 Sweet Strawberry Sugar Scrub

Strawberries are great for any girl, and it's a great body scrub for spring or summer. You'll find that freeze dried strawberries powder easily, and the antioxidants are great to keep you from feeling the effects of aging as harshly.

With coconut oil and almond oil for your skin, this is a wonderful sugar scrub.

Ingredients:

1. 1 ½ Cups Freeze Dried Strawberries
2. ¼ Cup Sweet Almond Oil
3. ¾ Cup Coconut Oil, Extra Virgin
4. 2 Cups White Sugar

Directions:

1. Start by powdering your freeze dried strawberries.
2. Mix all ingredients together, and place in an airtight glass container.

Body Scrub #45 Mint & Rosemary Sugar Scrub

Rosemary and mint is a relaxing and rejuvenating body scrub that will help you to feel better in both body and mind. Rosemary essential oil is relaxing, and it's also stimulating in a way, helping to calm your mind. Mint is also known to stimulate your senses while giving soothing relief.

Ingredients:

1. ¼ Cup Sea Salt, Fine
2. ¾ Cup White Sugar
3. 10-15 Drops Peppermint Essential Oil
4. 8-10 Drops Rosemary Essential Oil
5. 1 Teaspoon Rosemary, Dried
6. ½ Cup Sweet Almond Oil

Directions:

1. Just mix all ingredients together before you put it into your jar to decorate later.

Body Scrub #46 Vanilla Honey Body Scrub

Vanilla is full of antioxidants, and so is honey. It helps with aging, and it'll refresh and smooth out your skin in no time. It can even help with dry skin and acne, especially with the sweet almond oil added.

Ingredients:

1. ½ Cup Sweet Almond Oil
2. 1 Cup White Sugar
3. 2 Tablespoons Honey, Raw
4. 10-15 Drops Vanilla Essential Oil

Directions:

1. Just mix all ingredients together, making sure that the honey is mixed all the way through before putting it into a glass jar.

Body Scrub #47 Lemon & Orange Blossom Scrub

Lemon essential oil helps to firm up your skin and take away any oil that may be causing acne. With orange blossom essential oil added in the anti-inflammatory effects will make sure that your skin looks like new in no time, and it'll help to make sure that you have an uplifting scent to help with stress and anxiety.

Ingredients:

1. 1 Cup White Sugar
2. 10-15 Drops Orange Blossom Essential Oil
3. 8-10 Drops Lemon Essential Oil
4. ½ Cup Olive Oil

Directions:

1. Mix everything together, and then place in a container until you're ready to decorate and use or give as a gift.

Body Scrub #48 Spiced Brown Sugar Scrub

Brown sugar is a sweet and spiced blend that is sure to help you feel better and make you have softer skin in no time. You can use light brown sugar if you want, but make sure that all of your essential oils are mixed all the way through. Vanilla is uplifting, cinnamon is anti-inflammatory, and nutmeg is a great way to stop premature aging in its tracks.

Ingredients:

1. 1 Cup Brown Sugar, Dark & Packed
2. ½ Cup Sweet Almond Oil
3. 10-15 Drops Vanilla Essential Oil
4. 5-6 Drops Cinnamon Essential Oil
5. 2-4 Drops Nutmeg Essential Oil

Directions:

1. Mix everything together, making sure that your essential oils are mixed all the way through.

Body Scrub #49 Honeyed Ginger Body Scrub

Ginger and honey is always a good scent, and ginger essential oil is known to relax you, relieving any tension. Honey hydrates your skin and leaves it soft and moist, especially with coconut oil involved.

Ingredients:

1. 2 Tablespoons Honey, Raw
2. 10-12 Drops Ginger Essential Oil
3. ¼ Cup Sea Salt, Coarse
4. ¾ Cup White Sugar
5. ½ Cup Sweet Almond Oil

Directions:

1. Mix all ingredients together, making sure the honey is thoroughly mixed throughout.

Body Scrub #50 Grapefruit & Lemon Scrub

Grapefruit essential oils is known to help with depression, and it's even better for stress. Lemon is also known to help with stress, and it's a refreshing scent that will leave you feeling happy and your skin feeling soft.

Ingredients:

1. 8-10 Drops Grapefruit Essential Oil
2. 10-12 Drops Lemon Essential Oil
3. ½ Cup Coconut Oil, Melted
4. 1 Cup Sea Salt, Coarse

Directions:

1. Mix all ingredients together.

Some Final Tips:

You need some final tips to make sure that your gifts are they best they can be. Make sure to write a personal note, and you can even skip the card. If you have your scrubs layered, remember to say its fine to mix them all the way through if you want them to be perfect.

Men are Different: Men don't want to have a girly decorated body scrub with a manly scent. If you're looking to decorate a body scrub for a man, you may want to raid your garage and bring out the twine, duct tape, and washers. It's easy to make sure that you have what you need, and it doesn't have to be expensive. Keep it basic if nothing else, and don't go too frilly with the ribbon. Darker colors are usually best as well.

Burn the Edges: With ribbon, you don't want it to unravel. Hot glue will make sure it stays in place, but when you cut it into a nice point you're going to want a lighter to burn the edges. Just gently wave it underneath, and you should notice them burning, but don't let it catch on fire or curl. This will ruin the look and you'll need to start over.

Use the Right Pen: When you're hand writing things it seems a little more personal, so if you choose to handwrite your tags, make sure you're using the proper pen. Don't make it too bold or it might smear together, and too thin may make your handwriting seem a little weak. Use the color of your choice as well, but black or blue is always standard if you're looking for something classy. Of course, if you're going with a theme, feel free to mix the colors up.